Skin Health

A Comprehensive Guide To

Modern Dermatology

Dr. Clara Dermott

Contents

CHAPTER ONE

Introduction

One of the most effective drugs for the treatment and management of infections perpetrated by fungi is Ketoconazole. This amazing drug has proven over time in multiple medical situations to be efficient in permanently treating fungal diseases. It is available in diverse formulations to make it easier to use. It is available in cream, shampoo, and oral tablets.

The oral formulation can be taken with or without food, however, it should be taken after a diet to avoid ulcers and other gastrointestinal issues. The dose most appropriate for adults is 200mg every 24 hours, while kids below the age of 10 should be dosed based on their respective body weights.

The shampoo formulation is thoroughly massaged into the

hair and scalp specifically on the infected part to invite relief.

This formulation contains selenium sulfide; an active component that treats dandruff and seborrheic dermatitis.

This antifungal drug is highly recommended due to its

effectiveness in several fungal cases.

However, Ketoconazole can cause severe side effects affecting the liver and heart, and as such careful dosing and monitoring of the essence.

Every patient is advised to speak to a pharmacist or doctor before beginning usage.

How it works

Ketoconazole works by interfering with the growth process of the fungi causing the infection.

Ketoconazole hinders the fungi from synthesizing ergosterol; an active component of the cell membrane responsible for the growth of the fungi causing the infection.

This interference cures the infection by killing the organism causing the infection.

Alternative Medications and Natural Remedies

Ciclopirox is an antifungal medication as well, and can directly take the place of Ketoconazole. It can be used to cure infections affecting the nails and skin; particularly tinea versicolor, ringworm, and nail infections caused by fungi.

For the cure of ringworm and athlete's foot infections, Butenafine comes highly recommended. It is available in cream and gel varieties to enable convenience.

Econazole is another effective alternative for treating several fungal-related infections. It is available in cream and foam forms.

Coconut oil can be applied topically to eradicate any fungal infection on the skin.

For the treatment of jock itch? Terbinafine is the most effective antifungal alternative to Ketoconazole.

The Downsides of Topical Ketoconazole

The most common side effects associated with the usage of topical Ketoconazole are redness, itching, burning, and stinging of the treated or affected area of the skin.

Other patients may even be plagued with the drying peeling of their skin.

The Downsides of Oral Ketoconazole

The side effects associated with the oral form of Ketoconazole are mild and can be managed through dosage adjustments and other remedy alternatives.

Some patients may frequently feel the need to vomit and

experience severe pains in the abdominal regions. Liver problems are also a thing of worry when taking Ketoconazole, which is why careful monitoring and dosing are necessary during medication.

Unfortunately, Ketoconazole can also cause hormonal imbalance.

Using Ketoconazole can also result in the development of certain allergic reactions of the skin such as itching, swelling, drying, reddening, etc.

This medication can cause several side effects when combined or taken during the same duration as any other antifungal medication, supplements, or herbs. Such interactions could cause both medications to become ineffective.

CHAPTER TWO

The Dosing and Usage of Topical Ketoconazole

The topical formulation of Ketoconazole is available in 3 forms: Cream, foam, and Shampoo.

The cream form is to be applied once or twice daily on the

infected region of the skin, depending on the kind and severity of the infection or as instructed by your medical doctor.

For the treatment of hair and scalp-related infections like dandruff and dermatitis, wash the hair or scalp cleanly and then massage the formulation onto the infected area thoroughly. It is best recommended to do repeat this treatment procedure 3 or 4 times a week, or as instructed by your medical doctor or skincare specialist.

The foam form should be applied or massaged on the

affected area, the application

dosage and duration of

application depends on the

severity of the infection and the

instructions written on the

medication's label.

The duration of use of this

topical formulation will be

decided by the medical doctor

accessing the situation of your infection.

The Dosing of Oral Ketoconazole

The recommended starting dose for any adult is 200mg. The subsequent doses will be determined by the intensity of the infection and the response to the treatment.

Oral ketoconazole is always taken after a meal to reduce the risks of gastrointestinal side effects and increase the chances of absorption.

The duration of usage should be determined by a medical doctor after fully accessing your medical situation.

Necessary Precautions

One of the most significant precautions to take during the course of this medication is to ensure that the instructions given to you by a medical doctor are diligently adhered to. Take your medications as prescribed and ensure to complete the dosing even if the symptoms subside halfway. Completing your medication reduces the chances of the infection recurring.

Make sure you are under the medical watchfulness of a

professional doctor. Do not self-medicate.

Take your medications as prescribed by a medical doctor, do not skip or delay the intake of your doses.

Any patient using topical Ketoconazole should ensure to apply the cream or shampoo as frequently as instructed. Avoid skipping or delaying the prescribed periods of application.

Delaying or skipping your medications reduces the all-around effectiveness of the medication.

Avoid excessive application of the cream, or shampoo, and only apply them on the affected areas of the skin. Applying them to the unaffected areas will lead to unwanted skin irritations such as itching, burning, reddening, etc.

Interactions

Muscle-related issues can resurface if ketoconazole is used at the same time as medications such as Atorvastatin, and Simvastatin. These Statins are often used to minimize cholesterol and can cause serious muscle problems when taken in the same duration as Ketoconazole.

Ketoconazole doesn't interact friendly with anticoagulants such as warfarin. This combination can enhance the risk of bleeding.

Antacids have the properties to decrease the absorption of

Ketoconazole in the bloodstream.

Using Ketoconazole along with Digoxin can increase the risk of toxicity.

HIV medications are not friendly with Ketoconazole either. Hence, avoid using them during the same treatment phase.

When to speak to a medical doctor

Contact a medical doctor before using any formulations of Ketoconazole.

A medical professional will enable you to understand which is best for your kind of infection.

Do not switch to any Ketoconazole alternative without speaking to a medical professional first; to avoid unfriendly interactions.

Call the immediate attention of a medical doctor whenever you experience any of the aforementioned side effects associated with the use of

Ketoconazole.

THE END

www.ingramcontent.com/pod-product-compliance
Lightning Source LLC
Chambersburg PA
CBHW050709250726
48662CB00002B/922